HERBAL REMEDIES FOR MORNING SICKNESS

A Beginner's Guide To Discover Gentle And Effective Plant-Based Solutions To Ease Nausea And Embrace A Healthier Pregnancy Journey

DR. CHRIS FRIEDRICH

Disclaimer

This book on Herbal Remedies is intended solely for informational and educational purposes.

The content provided within this book is based on general knowledge and should not be considered as professional advice. The author is not a licensed medical professional, and the information presented here is not intended to diagnose, treat, cure, or prevent any disease.

Readers are advised to consult with qualified healthcare professionals before initiating any herbal remedies or making changes to their existing health regimen. The author and publisher disclaim any responsibility for any adverse effects or consequences resulting from the use of information contained in this book.

It's important to note that the content of this book is not endorsed by any specific platform or affiliated with any product or service. The author does not receive any compensation or benefits from the promotion of specific herbal products or brands.

Readers should exercise their discretion and judgment when applying the information from this book, and they are encouraged to conduct further research and seek guidance from healthcare professionals to make informed decisions about their health and well-being.

IMPORTANCE OF THIS BOOK

In-depth explanations of morning sickness' definition, symptoms, causes, and triggers are provided in "Herbal Remedies for Morning Sickness," a comprehensive guide to the long-standing practice of using herbal remedies to ease the discomfort associated with morning sickness during pregnancy. Through the integration of traditional wisdom and cultural practices, the reader is given important historical context for herbal remedies, which are enhanced by folklore passed down through the generations.

Its examination of herbal fundamentals forms the bulk of the book, systematically acquainting readers with the realm of herbal medicine. Safety recommendations and cautions are vital cornerstones that enable people to responsibly utilize the benefits of herbal remedies.

The chapters devoted to common morning sickness herbs—ginger, peppermint, and chamomile, for example—are priceless assets, delving into the qualities, applications, dosages, and methods of preparation of each herb, giving readers a firm basis upon which to implement these remedies in their daily lives.

The author's skill is evident in the section on creating herbal blends, which provides readers with synergistic combinations and DIY tea recipes. The book also addresses the various stages of pregnancy, offering specific herbal support for each trimester and extending its advice to postpartum care. Finally, the nutritional support section highlights the book's holistic approach by providing dietary guidelines and recipes infused with herbs to improve overall health.

The book's holistic approach is made clear as the story progresses, with yoga and meditation exercises tailored to morning sickness sufferers.

A separate chapter highlights the value of seeking medical advice from qualified healthcare providers and guides the judicious use of herbal remedies in prenatal care.

In-depth safety considerations are a major focus of the book, providing readers with relevant experiences, success stories, and priceless lessons learned on their herbal journey. Real-life stories and testimonials add a personal touch, illuminating herb-drug interactions, identifying which herbs to avoid during pregnancy, and encouraging an informed decision-making process.

"Herbal Remedies for Morning Sickness" is essentially more than just a list of remedies; it's a comprehensive manual that equips readers to safely, wisely, and confidently negotiate the complex terrain of pregnancy. As such, it's a priceless tool for expectant mothers looking for all-natural remedies for morning sickness.

CHAPTER I
UNDERSTANDING MORNING SICKNESS

Even though the term "morning sickness" refers to the nausea and vomiting that many pregnant women experiences, it can occur at any time of day. Morning sickness is a common pregnancy-related condition that affects a large number of women, albeit to varying degrees of severity.

Although the exact mechanisms underlying morning sickness are unknown, it is thought to be related to hormonal changes, specifically the increase in human chorionic gonadotropin (hCG) levels. Although morning sickness is generally accepted as a normal part of pregnancy, severe cases may need to be treated medically to manage symptoms and protect the developing fetus.

Meaning and Signs

Morning sickness is a term used to describe a variety of symptoms, the most common of which are nausea and vomiting.

Nausea is commonly defined as feeling queasy or wanting to throw up, while vomiting can occur occasionally or more frequently.

These symptoms can have a substantial negative influence on a pregnant person's quality of life and their capacity to go about their daily activities.

It is important to understand that morning sickness symptoms can vary greatly in severity and duration among pregnant women. Some may only have mild symptoms that go away after the first trimester, while others may suffer more intense and prolonged episodes of nausea and vomiting for the duration of their pregnancy.

Reasons and Initiators

Morning sickness has many different causes, including hormonal, physiological, and psychological factors.

The main cause of morning sickness is the increase in hCG levels, which are produced by the developing placenta. Other factors that contribute to the onset of symptoms are fluctuations in estrogen and progesterone levels; the precise interaction of these hormones and their effects on the gastrointestinal system is still being studied.

In addition to hormonal factors, some triggers can make morning sickness worse. These triggers can include sensitivity to certain smells, increased stress, and even pre-existing gastrointestinal conditions. Knowing these causes and triggers is essential for creating effective strategies to reduce and manage morning sickness.

Herbal Treatments for Morning Fatigue

In light of the desire to reduce exposure to medications during pregnancy, many people look into alternative and complementary ways to manage morning sickness. Herbal remedies have been a traditional way to treat pregnancy-related symptoms, but there is some variation in their efficacy, so caution should be used.

One commonly recommended herb is ginger, which has anti-nausea properties and can be consumed in tea, ginger ale, or ginger candies. Another herb is peppermint, which is thought to have soothing effects on the digestive system and can be consumed as tea or in aromatherapy. Although these herbal remedies may provide relief for some people, it's important to speak with a healthcare provider before incorporating them into a pregnancy wellness plan.

While morning sickness is a common pregnancy symptom that affects people differently, it's important to understand its underlying causes, symptoms and triggers to develop effective management strategies. Some pregnant women may find relief from morning sickness with herbal remedies like peppermint and ginger, but it's important to approach these options cautiously and consult with healthcare professionals to ensure safety and efficacy. Personal care is essential to supporting the well-being of both the expectant mother and the developing fetus.

CHAPTER 2
TRADITIONAL WISDOM

A rich tapestry of herbal remedies that reflect the diverse cultural perspectives on maternal health has been created over the years by communities around the world who have relied on the healing properties of plants to ease the discomfort associated with morning sickness during pregnancy. These communities have used herbal remedies for morning sickness for a long time, dating back many generations and cultures.

An Historical View on Herbal Medicines

The background of herbal remedies for morning sickness indicates how long people have relied on nature's abundance for medical purposes. Ancient Egyptians, Greeks, and Chinese were among the cultures that used a range of herbs to treat pregnancy's discomforts, which included nausea and vomiting.

Chinese traditional medicine records mention ginger and Greek texts emphasize the importance of peppermint and chamomile for calming the stomach. These historical customs highlight the persistent belief in the medicinal value of herbs for the health of mothers.

Cultural Customs and Legends

Many cultures place a strong emphasis on the holistic relationship between the pregnant woman and nature. For instance, in Ayurveda, an ancient Indian medical system, herbs like fennel and cardamom are believed to balance the doshas and promote overall well-being during pregnancy. Similarly, Native American traditions incorporate the use of herbal infusions, such as raspberry leaf tea, thought to strengthen the uterus and alleviate nausea. Herbal remedies for morning sickness are often embedded with cultural practices and folklore, reflecting the distinctive beliefs and customs of various communities.

Stories that have been passed down through the generations about wise women and herbalists who had access to secret plant-based remedy knowledge are common in the folklore surrounding herbal remedies for morning sickness.

For example, in European folklore, the use of herbs like peppermint and lemon balm is said to have been passed down through generations of midwives and herbal practitioners.

These kinds of stories add to the cultural significance of herbal remedies by encouraging a sense of continuity and trust in the efficacy of natural solutions.

Ultimately, the integration of traditional wisdom, historical context, cultural customs, and folklore offers a thorough comprehension of the function of herbal remedies in treating morning sickness in pregnancy.

The interaction of these components underscores the long-standing heritage of herbal knowledge in maternity healthcare and underscores the significance of honoring and conserving various cultural approaches to health.

CHAPTER 3
HERBAL BASICS

For centuries, herbal remedies have been a fundamental component of traditional medicine systems, providing a natural means of treating a wide range of ailments. In the case of morning sickness, a common ailment that affects pregnant women, herbal remedies have gained popularity due to their potential efficacy and low side effects; they are typically derived from plant sources and utilize the therapeutic properties of herbs to reduce morning sickness symptoms.

Overview of Herbal Medicine

Herbal medicine, sometimes referred to as phototherapy or botanical medicine, is the application of plants and plant extracts to treat and prevent disease. The practice has its roots in ancient civilizations when knowledge of herbs and their therapeutic qualities was passed down through the generations.

In the modern era, herbal medicine is still used as an adjunct or substitute for traditional medical treatments, with a focus on using the entire plant or specific parts of the plant, such as leaves, roots, or flowers, to harness a wide range of compounds that have healing properties.

Safety Instructions and Measures

Herbal remedies are often thought to be natural and safe, but it's important to use them carefully, especially when pregnant. Safety guidelines and precautions must be followed to protect the developing fetus as well as the mother.

Pregnant women should speak with their healthcare providers before using herbal remedies to avoid any negative effects or potential drug interactions. They should also closely monitor the dosage and duration of herbal treatments to avoid any unintended consequences.

To minimize the risks associated with herbal remedies, pregnant women should give priority to herbs that are generally recognized as safe during pregnancy and have a history of traditional use in supporting maternal well-being. Pregnant women should also be aware of the unique physiological changes that occur during pregnancy, as some herbs may stimulate uterine contractions or have hormonal effects.

Some herbs that may help with nausea management include peppermint and chamomile, but it's important to make sure you take them in forms that don't exceed recommended dosages. One well-researched herb with anti-nausea properties is ginger, which has been used historically to relieve morning sickness and is generally considered safe for pregnant women when consumed in moderate amounts.

While some herbs show promise in relieving symptoms, pregnant women must work closely with healthcare professionals to make informed decisions about the use of herbal remedies during pregnancy, ensuring the safety and well-being of both the mother and the unborn child.

Using herbal remedies in the management of morning sickness requires a nuanced understanding of herbal basics, the principles of herbal medicine, and strict adherence to safety guidelines and precautions.

CHAPTER 4
COMMON HERBS FOR MORNING SICKNESS

The active compounds in ginger, such as gingerol, contribute to its anti-nausea properties.

Ginger has long been known as nature's nausea reliever and is a popular herbal remedy for morning sickness. Its properties include antiemetic and anti-inflammatory effects, making it effective in alleviating nausea and vomiting. Ginger can be consumed in a variety of forms, such as fresh ginger root, ginger tea, or ginger supplements. Pregnant women often find relief by incorporating ginger into their diet, whether through ginger tea or by adding fresh ginger to meals. Nevertheless, it's important to speak with a healthcare provider to determine the right dosage for each patient.

Another herbal remedy that is well-known for its calming effects on the stomach is peppermint, which may also help with morning sickness.

The menthol in peppermint helps relax the muscles of the gastrointestinal tract, which lessens the symptoms of nausea. Peppermint can be inhaled or consumed as peppermint tea, though the latter should be used sparingly and diluted. Expectant mothers should speak with their healthcare providers before introducing peppermint into their routine to make sure it is appropriate for them.

As a calming effect on the digestive system, chamomile is especially useful for pregnant women who are experiencing morning sickness. Its anti-inflammatory and muscle-relaxant properties help to reduce nausea and discomfort.

One popular and gentle way to incorporate chamomile into a morning sickness relief routine is to make chamomile tea, but it's important to choose a high-quality, pregnancy-safe tea and follow recommended brewing guidelines.

Pregnant women should consult their healthcare provider before regularly consuming chamomile tea to ensure it is safe and appropriate for their pregnancy.

Herbal remedies for morning sickness can be found in addition to the aforementioned herbs. One such herb is lemon balm, which has calming properties and can be ingested as a tea or inhaled as an essential oil. However, caution and moderation are required, as excessive consumption of certain herbs may have unintended effects. Additionally, herbal remedies should not be used in place of medical advice, and pregnant women should consult their healthcare providers before introducing new herbs into their routine, especially if they are taking medications or have pre-existing health conditions. using herbal remedies for morning sickness should be done mindfully and under the supervision of a qualified healthcare professional.

CHAPTER 5
CRAFTING HERBAL BLENDS

Herbal remedies for morning sickness are made by combining a variety of herbs that are well-known for their anti-nausea and calming qualities.

For example, ginger, a popular remedy for nausea, can be blended with peppermint and chamomile to produce a calming and effective combination. Peppermint has a cooling effect, while chamomile eases the digestive tract.

The secret to making these herbal remedies for morning sickness is to recognize the synergistic effects of various herbs and to create a blend that specifically targets the needs of expectant mothers who are suffering from morning sickness.

Combined Effectively for Morning Sickness

The key to increasing the potency of herbal remedies for morning sickness is to combine herbs that work well together.

For instance, combining anti-nausea herbs like ginger and lemon balm with herbs that promote general health like nettle and raspberry leaf can result in a well-rounded blend; nettle is high in vitamins and minerals, and raspberry leaf has a toning effect on the uterus. By carefully choosing complementary herbs, a holistic remedy that not only relieves nausea but also offers nutritional support during pregnancy can be made.

DIY Recipes for Herbal Tea:

A simple but effective tea can be made by steeping grated ginger, a few peppermint leaves, and chamomile flowers in hot water; this calming mixture can be sweetened with honey and sipped throughout the day. Another way to make a morning sickness remedy is to combine herbs like lemon balm and spearmint with a little lemon zest to create a refreshing tea that helps alleviate nausea. DIY herbal tea recipes enable people to experiment with different herbs, adjusting ratios to find the most comforting and effective blend for their morning sickness relief.

Using Aromatherapy to Reduce Nausea

A non-invasive and enjoyable way for pregnant women to manage morning sickness symptoms is aromatherapy for nausea relief. Aromatherapy uses essential oils such as ginger, peppermint, and lemon. Inhaling the aroma of ginger essential oil, for example, has been shown to have anti-nausea effects. Diffusing peppermint oil in the living space or inhaling its scent directly can provide a refreshing and soothing experience.

Lemon essential oil, with its uplifting fragrance, not only helps combat nausea but also contributes to a positive mood.

When used in aromatherapy, essential oils like ginger, lemon, and peppermint can be included.

The ideas behind creating herbal blends, synergistically combining herbs, making herbal tea at home, and using aromatherapy to reduce nausea provide a variety of approaches to treating morning sickness. Through knowledge of the characteristics of different herbs and how they work together, people can customize remedies to suit their tastes and circumstances, creating a more comprehensive and individualized method of addressing the difficulties associated with morning sickness in pregnancy.

CHAPTER 6
HERBS FOR DIFFERENT STAGES OF PREGNANCY

First Trimester Remedies: Morning sickness is a common concern for many women during the first trimester of pregnancy. Herbal remedies can help during this delicate period. For example, ginger has been known for its anti-nausea properties; ginger tea or capsules can be useful in reducing nausea and settling an upset stomach.

Also, because peppermint and lemon balm teas have calming effects on the digestive system, they may be helpful. These herbs can be consumed in tea form or added to meals to help manage morning sickness symptoms without the need for prescription drugs.

Considerations for the Second and Third Trimesters: During the second and third trimesters of pregnancy, some herbs can still be helpful.

One popular option is raspberry leaf tea, which is thought to help tone the uterine muscles and get the body ready for labor. However, before implementing any herbal remedies, especially in the later stages of pregnancy, it is important to speak with a healthcare professional.

Nettle tea is another herbal option that is rich in essential nutrients like iron, which can be helpful for pregnant women. These herbs can benefit the mother and the growing child when used carefully and moderately.

Postpartum Herbal Support: Following childbirth, herbal remedies can still be beneficial in aiding the postpartum healing process. Herbs like fenugreek and fennel are frequently used to help nursing mothers produce milk. Chamomile and lavender teas can calm and relax new mothers, assisting them in managing the physical and mental strain of the postpartum phase. Nursing mothers need to be aware of the herbs they take, as some may impact the milk supply or be transferred to the baby through breast milk.

Consulting with a qualified healthcare provider is advised to guarantee the safety and effectiveness of herbal remedies during the postpartum period.

Ultimately, herbal remedies can be helpful allies in the management of morning sickness and in supporting the various stages of pregnancy.

However, expectant mothers must speak with their healthcare providers before implementing any herbal treatments into their routine, as each person's body reacts differently to herbs and a healthcare professional can provide customized advice based on the unique needs and circumstances of the pregnancy.

Incorporating herbal remedies sensibly and under professional guidance can improve the general health of the expectant mother as well as the developing baby for the duration of the pregnancy as well as the postpartum period.

CHAPTER
NUTRITIONAL SUPPORT

The key to using herbal remedies for morning sickness is nutritional support.

A woman's nutritional needs are increased during pregnancy, and some herbs can supply vital vitamins and minerals. Herbs like peppermint and ginger can reduce nausea and promote digestive health; adding these herbs to the diet can offer a natural and comprehensive method of nutritional support during pregnancy.

Diet and Nutrition for Morning Sickness: Diet is a key component in treating morning sickness, and including herbal remedies in daily consumption can be helpful. One such herb is ginger, which has been extensively researched for its anti-nausea effects. Drinking ginger tea or adding fresh ginger to meals can help reduce nausea and enhance overall digestion.

Another useful herb is peppermint, which can be added to the diet to relieve morning sickness symptoms.

Finally, a well-balanced diet that incorporates these herbal elements can help the expectant mother's general health.

Pregnancy-Friendly Herbal Infusion Recipes: Pregnancy-friendly herbal infusions can be a fun and efficient way for a pregnant woman to incorporate herbal remedies into her daily routine. Chamomile or lemon balm herbal teas can be calming and aid with nausea.

Lemon balm, which has calming properties, can be added to salad recipes or infused water. Dandelion greens, which are high in nutrients, can be added to salads or smoothies to boost the nutritional value of meals. Using these herbal ingredients in recipes not only offers a delicious culinary experience but also helps manage morning sickness healthfully and naturally.

It is important to remember that although herbal remedies have their uses, expectant mothers should speak with their healthcare provider before making major dietary changes or adding new herbs to their regimen. Every pregnancy is different, and seeking professional advice guarantees the mother's safety and the health of the unborn child.

HOLISTIC APPROACHES

Herbal remedies play a significant role in holistic approaches to morning sickness management because they are often considered natural and gentle alternatives to conventional medications. By promoting overall health and bringing the body's systems into harmony, herbal remedies may be able to alleviate morning sickness symptoms without causing harmful side effects. Holistic approaches to managing morning sickness involve treating the individual rather than just the symptoms.

Mind-Body Link

A key component of holistic health is the mind-body connection, which highlights the relationship between mental and physical health.

Stress and anxiety can aggravate morning sickness symptoms, and herbal remedies, which have calming effects, attempt to address both the mind and the body. Adding relaxation techniques, like deep breathing and mindfulness, into daily routines can support herbal interventions.

By addressing the mind-body connection, people may see a decrease in the intensity and frequency of morning sickness symptoms, promoting a more balanced state of well-being.

Meditation and Yoga to Treat Morning Sickness

Together, yoga, meditation, and herbal remedies form a synergistic approach that addresses the physical and mental aspects of morning sickness, offering a holistic pathway to relief.

Specific yoga poses may help alleviate digestive discomfort and promote relaxation, while meditation can serve as a mental anchor during moments of nausea.

Yoga and meditation are powerful tools in the holistic management of morning sickness because they emphasize gentle movements, controlled breathing, and mental centering.

Herbal remedies can further enhance the calming and anti-nausea effects of these practices.

While many people with morning sickness find relief from their symptoms with herbal remedies, yoga, and meditation, it is imperative to speak with a healthcare provider before beginning any new practice, especially during pregnancy, as every person's body responds differently and personalized guidance ensures the safety and appropriateness of these holistic approaches.

Keeping the lines of communication open with healthcare providers also enables a comprehensive approach to managing morning sickness that combines conventional and alternative methods for optimal well-being.

CONSULTING WITH HEALTHCARE PROFESSIONALS

Healthcare professionals, such as obstetricians, midwives, or herbalists, can offer personalized advice based on your medical history and ensure the safety of both you and your developing baby. While herbal remedies can be considered a natural approach to managing morning sickness, it is important to ensure that they do not pose any risks or contraindications to your particular health condition or pregnancy before incorporating them into your prenatal care routine.

Including Herbal Treatments in Prenatal Healthcare

Herbal remedies should be introduced into prenatal care with caution because pregnancy is a delicate time, and any changes to your routine should be carefully considered. Choosing to incorporate herbal remedies into prenatal care requires careful consideration and thoughtful decision-making; it is best to begin with small doses and observe how your body reacts, keeping an eye out for any negative effects. Furthermore, herbal remedies should be used in addition to, not in place of, traditional prenatal care practices like regular check-ups and proper nutrition.

Talking with Your Healthcare Provider About Herbal Options

When it comes to herbal remedies for morning sickness, it is important to communicate with your healthcare provider. Having an open line of communication allows them to be aware of any supplements or herbs they are taking, which enables them to provide guidance and watch out for potential drug interactions.

Your provider can also assist you in making decisions about which herbs to take, how much of them to take, and any possible side effects. This cooperative approach guarantees that your pregnancy journey is supported and that any herbal remedies you choose are in line with the overall objectives of your prenatal care plan.

Herbal remedies are a useful addition to treating morning sickness, but they are not a one-size-fits-all solution. People respond differently to herbal supplements, and what works for one person may not work for another. For this reason, it's critical to have open and continuous communication with your healthcare provider to customize your herbal regimen to your particular needs and situation.

In summary, incorporating herbal remedies into prenatal care for morning sickness necessitates careful thought and cooperation with medical professionals. You can safely and effectively navigate the use of herbal supplements during pregnancy by speaking with your healthcare provider, integrating remedies thoughtfully, and keeping lines of communication open. You should always put your health and the health of your unborn child first, pay close attention to any changes in your health, and seek professional advice as soon as necessary.

CHAPTER 6
SAFETY AND CONTRAINDICATIONS

When thinking about using herbal remedies for morning sickness while pregnant, it's important to focus on safety and be mindful of any possible contraindications. Women who are expecting should proceed with caution and seek medical advice before introducing herbal remedies into their regimen. Safety is important because some herbs can be harmful to the mother and the growing fetus. It's also important to remember that each person reacts differently to different herbs, so it's important to use herbal remedies with caution.

Recognizing Drug-Herb Interactions

Herbal-drug interactions are an important factor to take into account when researching herbal remedies for morning sickness.

Certain herbs can cause problems with the way prescription medications are absorbed, metabolized, or worked. Pregnant women should let their healthcare providers know about any herbal supplements they are thinking about so that any potential interactions can be thoroughly assessed. Herbalists and medical professionals working together can help develop a safe and comprehensive treatment plan.

Which Herbs Are Safe to Take During Pregnancy?

Some herbs are contraindicated in pregnancy because they may harm the developing fetus or interfere with normal physiological processes. Certain herbs should be used cautiously or not at all if you have morning sickness. Some of these herbs are pennyroyal, tansy, and juniper; these herbs have been known to have emmenagogue properties, which means they may stimulate menstruation and harm the pregnancy. Other herbs, like black cohosh and blue cohosh, may stimulate the uterus and should be avoided during pregnancy.

To sum up, safety concerns and knowing which herbs to avoid while pregnant are essential when researching herbal remedies for morning sickness. Expectant mothers should prioritize talking to healthcare providers, investigate possible drug interactions, and choose herbs carefully to protect the developing fetus as well as the mother.

CHAPTER 7
REAL-LIFE STORIES AND TESTIMONIALS

Testimonials and anecdotes from people who have used herbal remedies for morning sickness provide important context for understanding how effective these natural treatments are. People who have personally dealt with the difficulties of morning sickness frequently share their experiences, which throws light on the various ways that herbal remedies have helped to manage or alleviate symptoms. These personal accounts give the conversation a human face and help others relate to the practical and emotional benefits of incorporating herbal solutions into their pregnancy journeys.

Experiences with herbal remedies for morning sickness are widely varied, reflecting the individuality of each person's body and the particular nature of their symptoms.

Mothers-to-be can share their stories about how different herbs, like ginger, peppermint, or chamomile, have affected their health during pregnancy; these accounts often emphasize the value of customized approaches because what works for one person may not work for another. The examination of these varied experiences adds to a collective body of knowledge that enables people to make well-informed decisions about integrating herbal remedies into their morning sickness management plans.

A ray of hope for those looking for complementary and alternative methods to treat morning sickness symptoms are success stories involving the use of herbal remedies. These stories typically highlight the benefits and relief that people who have incorporated herbs into their daily routines have experienced, and learning about the elements that made a success—such as the particular herbs used, dosage, and consistency—can be helpful to others who are contemplating a similar course of action. Finally, these success stories serve as inspiration for expectant mothers to investigate herbal remedies under the supervision of medical professionals and include them in their overall wellness regimens.

The experiences of expectant mothers provide valuable insights into potential pitfalls, challenges, and unanticipated outcomes that they encountered when using herbal remedies for morning sickness. These insights can help others make informed decisions and encourage mindfulness and responsibility when incorporating herbal remedies into their prenatal care routines.

Some of the lessons learned from personal experiences and success stories include consulting with healthcare providers, considering individual sensitivities, and realizing the complementary nature of herbal remedies alongside conventional medical interventions.

Testimonials and real-life accounts weave a rich tapestry of insights into the world of herbal remedies for morning sickness.

Firsthand accounts provide a nuanced understanding of the various ways in which people have incorporated herbs into their pregnancy journeys. Success stories demonstrate the beneficial effects of herbal remedies when used sparingly. Takeaways add to a body of knowledge that promotes a well-rounded and educated approach, enabling expectant mothers to make decisions that are in line with their particular needs and circumstances.

CONCLUSION

While traditional medical interventions are available, there is a growing interest in investigating herbal remedies as alternative options. Herbal wisdom, derived from centuries-old practices, offers a holistic approach to managing morning sickness. Knowing the principles underlying herbal remedies for morning sickness can empower mothers to make choices that will lead to a healthier pregnancy.

Morning sickness is a common occurrence during pregnancy and can be a challenging experience for many expectant mothers.

Herbal Customs and Cultural Understanding

Traditional herbalists frequently incorporate locally available plants and herbs, taking into account not only their physiological effects but also their cultural significance. This intersection of tradition and culture contributes to a rich tapestry of herbal remedies that have stood the test of time. Throughout the world, diverse cultures have relied on the knowledge passed down through generations to address pregnancy-related discomforts.

The Variety of Plants and Active Ingredients

The key to the efficacy of herbal remedies is their variety of botanical sources and active compounds. For instance, ginger has been a well-liked option because of its anti-nausea properties; the active compounds, like gingerol, work with the body's systems to relieve symptoms. Other herbs that are well-known for their calming effects on the digestive system include peppermint, chamomile, and lemon balm. Mothers can select appropriate herbal remedies by knowing the botanical diversity and the specific compounds that are responsible for the therapeutic effects.

Safety Observations and Discussion

Herbal remedies are a natural alternative, but there are important safety considerations to be aware of when using them during pregnancy.

Not all herbs are safe for pregnant women, and they should be carefully evaluated for any potential interactions with conventional medications. Speaking with a healthcare professional—preferably one with experience in herbal medicine—becomes essential to ensuring that any herbal remedy selected is in line with the patient's health profile and minimizes risks to the mother and unborn child.

Lifestyle and Holistic Wellness Factors

Herbal remedies are frequently used in conjunction with a more comprehensive approach to holistic wellness during pregnancy.

Lifestyle factors, such as nutrition, exercise, and stress management, are important in reducing morning sickness. By incorporating herbal remedies into a holistic wellness plan, mothers can address the underlying causes of discomfort and enhance their overall well-being.

The use of herbal remedies is enhanced by an emphasis on a balanced lifestyle, which also helps to create a healthier pregnancy experience.

Empowerment via Knowledgeable Decisions

Since every woman's pregnancy journey is different, empowering mothers with herbal wisdom means giving them the knowledge and resources they need to make educated decisions. Educating them about botanical diversity, cultural insights, herbal remedies, safety considerations, and holistic wellness all contribute to a sense of empowerment that allows mothers to actively participate in their healthcare decisions and make decisions that are in line with their values and preferences.

This empowerment goes beyond treating morning sickness and lays the groundwork for a proactive and positive approach to overall maternal health.

Ultimately, investigating herbal remedies for morning sickness represents a comprehensive strategy for pregnancy wellness, extending beyond the pursuit of physical comfort. By utilizing the diverse range of herbal traditions, appreciating botanical diversity, taking professional guidance into account for safety, and adopting holistic lifestyle elements, one can become an informed and empowered mother on her journey.

When anticipating a healthy pregnancy, the incorporation of herbal knowledge proves to be an invaluable ally, offering not only morning sickness relief but also a more profound relationship with the ancient knowledge that has guided generations of mothers.